50 THINGS TO KNOW ABOUT FEMALE HEALTH, BEAUTY AND HYGIENE

GUIDE TO A BETTER LIFE

MUNEEBA ANWAR

iii

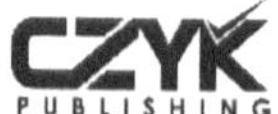

CZYK Publishing Since 2011.

50 Things to Know
Visit our website at www.50thingstoknow..com

Lock Haven, PA
All rights reserved.
ISBN: 9781790914289

50 THINGS TO KNOW
BOOK SERIES
REVIEWS FROM READERS

I recently downloaded a couple of books from this series to read over the weekend thinking I would read just one or two. However, I so loved the books that I read all the six books I had downloaded in one go and ended up downloading a few more today. Written by different authors, the books offer practical advice on how you can perform or achieve certain goals in life, which in this case is how to have a better life.

The information is simple to digest and learn from, and is incredibly useful. There are also resources listed at the end of the book that you can use to get more information.

50 Things To Know To Have A Better Life: Self-Improvement Made Easy! by Dannii Cohen

---

This book is very helpful and provides simple tips on how to improve your everyday life. I found it to be useful in improving my overall attitude.

50 Things to Know For Your Mindfulness & Meditation Journey by Nina Edmondso

---

Quick read with 50 short and easy tips for what to think about before starting to homeschool.

50 Things to Know About Getting Started with Homeschool by Amanda Walton

I really enjoyed the voice of the narrator, she speaks in a soothing tone. The book is a really great reminder of things we might have known we could do during stressful times, but forgot over the years.

-    HarmonyHawaii

50 Things to Know to Manage Your Stress: Relieve The Pressure and Return The Joy To Your Life

by Diane Whitbeck

There is so much waste in our society today. Everyone should be forced to read this book. I know I am passing it on to my family.

50 Things to Know to Downsize Your Life: How To Downsize, Organize, And Get Back to Basics

by Lisa Rusczyk Ed. D.

Great book to get you motivated and understand why you may be losing motivation. Great for that person who wants to start getting healthy, or just for you when you need motivation while having an established workout routine.

50 Things To Know To Stick With A Workout: Motivational Tips To Start The New You Today

by Sarah Hughes

50 THINGS TO KNOW ABOUT FEMALE HEALTH, BEAUTY AND HYGIENE

BOOK DESCRIPTION

Do you wish to explore your sexuality?

Are you seeking ways to improve your feminine health?

How can you become prettier naturally?

If you answered yes to any of these questions then this book is for you...

50 things to know about female health, hygiene and beauty by Muneeba Anwar offers an approach to choosing the right ways to improve your physical and sexual wellbeing. Most books on female health and hygiene will tell you only about the issues relating to it but not the solutions. Although there's nothing wrong with that but having a list of ways to improve the situation and remedies will help you a lot. Based on knowledge from the practicing pharmacist and a medical writer, this book will provide you deeper insights of health and hygiene issues that women experience in their day to day life.

In these pages you'll discover how essential and at the same time, easy it is to maintain your health and hygiene. This book will help you discover more about the needs of your body and how to fulfill them.

By the time you finish this book, you will know which natural ingredients and food items are your best friends and what to avoid when it comes to a being beautiful and healthy. So, grab YOUR copy today. You'll be glad you did.

TABLE OF CONTENTS

16. Probiotics Are Your Best Friend!

17. Nail Your Wiping Technique

18. Avoid Soap To Maintain PH Balance

19. Brush Your Tongue

20. Let's Wear Cotton Underwear

21. Treat Infections When They Arise

22. Use Enough Lubricant, but Not Petroleum Jelly

23. Eating And Hygiene

24. Urinate After Sex

25. Include More Yogurt In Your Diet

26. Get Regular Testing For STDs

27. Mild Soaps To Wash The Breast Area

28. Consider Taking Liquid Chlorophyll

29. Floss!

30. Get To Know Your Vaginal Scent

31. Correct Cleanser For Your Skin Type

32. Gentle Exfoliation Twice A Week

33. Stay Hydrated

34. Get Enough Sleep

35. Make Sunscreens Your Best Friend

36. Moisturizing Your Skin

37. Hair Care Routine

38. Eat Your Greens!

39. Green Tea For Weight Loss

40. Dark Colored Undergarments and Cancer

41. Dealing With The After-effects Of Vaginal Birth

DEDICATION

This book is affectionately dedicated to my parents, sister Asma and fiancé Hamid Raza.

ABOUT THE AUTHOR

I'm a licensed pharmacist and a medical writer. I have completed my PHARM-D degree from University of Central Punjab, Pakistan. I'm passionate about medical writing and researching.

If you wish to know more about me and contact me then here are the links:

https://www.linkedin.com/in/muneeba-anwar
https://www.upwork.com/fl/muneebaanwar22

INTRODUCTION

"If you really want to change the culture to empower women improve basic hygiene and health care and fight high rates of infant mortality the answer is to educate girls"

Greg Mortenson

Women have to maintain their health, hygiene and beauty along with their hectic jobs, studies and kids too. Sometimes very small issues related to their health and hygiene can lead to serious problems if they are left unattended.

This book covers small and pesky issues related to sexual health and hygiene, beauty and physical well-being. It also includes basic home remedies to deal with such problems. The goal is to educate women and empower them by letting them know that they have a total control over body and health.

The inspiration of writing this book came from a lot of ladies around me who keep asking me for easy solutions for their everyday problems. Being a pharmacist and a medical writer, I tried to gather all the information and summarized them for you. I hope my knowledge can prove helpful for you.

1.   ALWAYS SMELL GOOD!

One of the most important things which determine how you are going to be perceived by others is decided by how you smell. Humans have a natural tendency towards scented things like flowers, perfumes, natural body aromas and more. Have you ever wondered why wearing the same socks you wore yesterday makes you feel uncomfortable in public? Or not wearing your signature scent makes you feel that you're naked? This is because you assume that you're not smelling good and others are also noticing it!!

Just before or immediately after your special monthly days, most of the girls complain that they are sick of fishy smell that comes with thick white discharge. You should know that every vagina smells bad to a certain extent but If it exceeds that certain level and starts to smell like a dead fish! WARNING!! You might have some bacterial or yeast infection. Oh no! You don't have to panic about it.

Here are few simple tips to keep everything smelling nice and healthy – wear dry and light underwear all the time, avoid using scented products like fancy soaps and creams down there because they cause PH of the vagina to increase. Increased vaginal PH allows strict and harmful bacteria to grow in numbers, resulting in infections and ultimately that fishy smell.

Next, you can use natural oils like lavender and peppermint oil, and rub it directly on your lower belly and gently massage it down there. It will not only make you smell awesome but will soothe your muscles and vessels down there, maintaining a healthy flow of blood.

2.   KEEP EVERYTHING DRY!

Do you like exercising and swimming? If your answer is yes, then it is also likely that you are not taking the necessary measures after a healthy 30 minutes or more session. Most of us are so lazy that we sit at the edge of the pool talking to our friends or we just gossip about how much weight the other girl has lost, instead of taking a shower and changing fresh and dry clothes afterward.

The problem with wet clothes and undergarments is that they provide an ideal environment for the harmful bacteria and yeast to grow. Bacteria and yeast love to reside in an environment which is humid, moist, and warm. The problem doesn't end there, with an increased number of micro-organism comes increased chances of getting an infection or disease or in other words discomfort, itching, inflammation, smelly discharge, and more complications.

In order to maintain healthy and hygienic environment down there firstly wear cotton underpants, secondly change your clothes immediately after exercising and swimming or any other such activity which involves getting wet, thirdly wash properly and dry your girly parts after having sex or shower.

3.   ALLOW ALL YOUR BODY TO BREATHE!

Have you ever wondered why yoga instructors or health gurus ask you to breathe deeply? I mean like breathing is breathing, deep or shallow, what difference does that make? Well! Deep breathing allows every single cell of your body to bathe in the nourishing pool of oxygen-rich blood, sending the sensation of alertness and calmness throughout the body and you feel refreshingly better.

Just like you need to take in air to stay alive and active, your skin needs it too!! You cannot keep your skin covered in layers of tight clothing items. For instance, if you keep your vagina covered with tight underwear made of silk thread or nylon especially during the times of high humidity, you are extremely prone to developing an infection down there because they lock moisture and heat and the fact that bacteria and yeast love to reside in humid regions. Therefore, you have to make sure you keep it light down there by wearing undergarments which are made of cotton. Cotton allows proper ventilation and keeps the skin young and free from infections, absorbs unnecessary moisture and stops the unwanted odor.

4. AVOID USING BEAUTY PRODUCTS DOWN THERE

With ever-increasing advancements in technology and digital media, more and more people are getting attracted to buy and use all those fancy products available in the market, claiming to beautify and solve all your problems just like that.

Some of the claims might be true but the problem is not with what they claim, the problem is with what they contain! They contain harsh chemicals which can cause itching, PH imbalance, rash, and allergies.

So, how are you going to clean your vagina?

First of all, you need to get your facts straight! You do not need to clean your vagina, it's the vulva-

external part of the vagina that needs cleaning. The vagina is capable of self-cleaning and it maintains its PH with the help of healthy acid secreting Lactobacilli. When you use chemical containing soaps, shampoo, creams or moisturizers, they disrupt the PH balance causing it to become basic. PH above 4.5 provides ideal conditions for the growth of bacteria, ultimately infections and rash.

So, in order to clean the external parts of your genitalia simply take a soft loofah and water for gentle rinsing and exfoliation. You can also add a few drops of lavender oil in the water that will make everything smell like lavenders if that's what you wish.

5. DEAL WITH YOUR MENSTRUAL PAIN LIKE A BOSS!

Most of the girls nowadays complain about suffering from serious cramps and pain, starting a few days before your periods and continuing throughout the periods. This can affect your daily chores, mood, and social life. Nobody wants to suffer from pain while everybody else is just going out, partying and more. This pain is normally referred to as "dysmenorrhea" and occurs because of the hormone-like chemical –

prostaglandins when they try to shed the endometrial lining of the uterus by contracting.

Here are some of the tips and tricks to get rid of these cramps and pain.

The first thing you need to do is to stay away from cold things especially ice-creams, cold juices, drinks and make sure you stay covered and warm. Second most important thing is to add healthy food items in your diets such as green tea, garlic, boiled eggs and more because they can keep your vessels dilated and allow the blood to freely flow out of your body without clogging.

Next, if you're a big fan of coffee and tea just try to reduce the intake of these drinks because they might be warm but they have caffeine which constricts your vessel and you can imagine how it will pain when blood full off clots and shredded pieces of our internal lining will try to flow out of these constricted vessels.

For the next tip, I would like to introduce every mother's favorite remedy also known as a hot water bag. Yes! This little rubber bag filled with water can work like wonders when it comes to getting rid of cramps and pain. Just add some warm water into it and place it on your lower belly, make sure that it's not too hot, just enough to soothe your body muscles and you're good to go.

6. MENSTRUAL RASH? NOT A PROBLEM ANYMORE

Not many of us suffer from rashes and itching problems now, during menstruation days. Thanks to all these campaigns and ads that keep us aware of how to maintain healthy hygiene and use quality products. Some of us are still learning and trying to fight with menstrual rashes and itching. That may not be because they are not maintaining their hygiene or using low-grade products but it may be due to their extra sensitive skin.

If that's the case with you, then you need to go an extra mile to make sure that you don't get these rashes during your days because cramps, pain, and discomfort are already enough to make us curse ourselves.

To avoid these rashes, I've gathered a few tips for you. First of all, maybe by hit and trial or because you're knowledgeable enough unlike me, make sure to use sanitary pads that doesn't irritate your skin type. Next step is to wear loose clothing and allow your skin to breathe as I've mentioned earlier. If your skin is dry and scaly already then try drinking as much water as you can to keep it hydrated. If that doesn't do the trick then you can simply go for some anti-rash cream or natural oils. Just make sure that it's not damp or tight down there. Because that'll increase

friction while you walk or do your work and you'll
end up getting rashes.

## 7.	DO YOU SUFFER FROM PRE-MENSTRUAL SYNDROME?

As the name suggests, a sudden change in physical
health, emotional well-being, and behaviors just
before the menstrual days is referred to as a Pre-
menstrual syndrome or PMS. More than 80% of
women experience PMS symptoms before and during
their periods. These are more common in the women
of childbearing age. Symptoms might include acne
bursts, anxiety, depression, mood swings, cravings for
certain types of food, feeling fatigued and lethargic,
weight gain or loss and last but not the least severe
headaches and insomnia.

If you can relate to the occurrence of few or all of
these symptoms mentioned above that too just before
your periods, then you really need to step up your
game and deal with it like a pro. It is highly
recommended to increase your water intake that will
help you fight with acne bursts to a certain extent.
Calcium supplements and iron supplements reduce
the feeling of tiredness and lethargy. Similarly, for
your mood swings and anxiety, try adding stress
management programs in your life. Exercises such as

aerobics, cycling, and walking also help a great deal in stress management.

8.   AVOID TAKING ANTIBIOTICS

Antibiotics are the medicines that are supposed to kill all the pathogenic bacteria when you're suffering from any acute infections and diseases. No doubt, they're very efficacious and relieve symptoms and severity of the disease very quickly.

The problem with having them too often is that they can also kill your good bacteria present in your gut, on your skin or in your vagina. Once your good bacteria reduce in number the whole system goes out of order because antibiotics can't make good bacteria recolonize. In that case, taking antibiotics for reducing the symptoms of one infection can lead to other infections or recurrence of the same infection. Vaginal infections such as Bacterial Vaginosis or Yeast infections should be treated with probiotics and natural things such as cranberry or elderberry extracts. Even if the case is as such that taking antibiotics is inevitable, make sure to add probiotics to your diet right away.

9.   UNUSUAL WEIGHT GAIN

You might have experienced unusual weight gain at some point in your life or you might have seen someone complaining about it. There are several reasons why your weight is increasing even though you are not doing anything to make the scale go crazy. Let's break down a few of the reasons for you to understand that it's not something unusual rather it's the result of you being careless about your routine. Firstly, if you stay up till late at night you might opt for eating unhealthy snacks while binge-watching your favorite seasons or shows. Sleep deprivation might add to your suffering because it makes your body go out of hormonal balance which ultimately increases your appetite and hunger.

Stress also plays its part when it comes to the unusual increase in your weight. This is because of the fact that under the conditions of stress and anxiety your body releases a hormone called "cortisol". Cortisol is basically a stress hormone which also tends to increase your appetite, therefore, chronic stress results in unusual weight gain too.

Medications including antipsychotics, drugs for migraines, seizures, diabetes, blood pressure, and antidepressants are also considered to be the triggers of unusual weight gain. You have to make sure that you're not taking any medication without a prescription and that you have to report any unusual change immediately to your doctor.

10. BLEMISHES, DARK SPOTS, AND PIMPLES!

Have you ever got sudden burst out of pimples or acne and that too when your most awaited event or party is coming up? I know, most of the girls out there can relate. Even though it's extremely stressful but what's more hassling is the fact that these pimples or acne might leave scars, dead skin and uneven skin tone behind. This is where your mum's natural remedies will come handy to you.

Take yogurt, gram flour, and turmeric powder and mix them well. Apply them on your face at least 2-3 times a week. Leave it on for 20 minutes then rinse properly. Antioxidant and anti-inflammatory properties of turmeric and gram flour will help you get rid of blemishes and yogurt will moisturize your skin and give it a cooling effect. Tomatoes have antioxidant properties and vitamin C in them, which makes it an ideal remedy for removing tan and blemishes. Make sure that you apply sunscreen every single time when you go out in the sun because sun rays can trigger the production of melanin. Melanin is the chemical responsible for the dark color of the skin. Essential oils such as lavender and tea tree oils have strong antioxidant and skin rejuvenating properties. Applying them on your face twice or thrice a week and leaving them on whole night helps in reducing the blemishes and dark spots.

Last but not least, the potato can also be used to lighten the tone of the skin and make it even because of its bleaching actions. Take a potato and grate it, add few drops of lemon and apply it on the affected parts of your face, leave this paste on for 10-15 minutes and rinse your face properly.

11.   APPLE CIDER VINEGAR- A BLESSING IN DISGUISE

Even though the apple cider vinegar is being utilized for various purposes from centuries but its usage as a health and beauty enhancing product is now becoming popular worldwide. Not only its benefits are proven by myths and experiments but they are also backed by scientific research. Some of the most common health and beauty benefits include weight loss, reduced cholesterol level, balanced blood sugar, treatment and prevention of bacterial and fungal infections, hair conditioner, nail strengthening effects, skin lightening, and skin healing masks.

Drinking 1-2 tablespoons of organic apple cider vinegar diluted with water just before the meals will help you control your gut health, improves digestion and maintains a healthy blood sugar level after the meal. If you are suffering from recurring vaginal infections or fungal infections on your feet, then it's high time that you opt for this wonder ingredient. You can fill your bathtub with lukewarm water and add apple cider vinegar to it, allow your body to soak in it for at least half an hour. This will kill all the harmful bacteria and fungus present on your skin or in your vagina.

12.   INGROWN – AN ITCHY ISSUE

If you don't know already, those tiny bumps on your face or vagina which don't even look like a pimple or hive are actually ingrown hair. They're actually that hair which refuses to grow out normally like others rather they curl up and grow back into the skin. They appear mostly after waxing, shaving or tweezing, especially, when you have cut them too close to the skin. Girls who have more thick or curly hair are more likely to have ingrown hairs.

They are extremely itchy and annoying and above that, they have a tiny pimple or red bumpy appearance. In women, they mostly grow around the legs, armpits or pubic area. Generally, there is no specific treatment for ingrown hair but you can surely prevent them.

You should gently scrub or exfoliate your skin in a circular motion every day. Make sure to wash the area you're about to shave or wax with lukewarm water and use a sharp razor. Avoid multiple razor strokes and don't shave too close to the skin. Lastly, apply cold press or a cool wet cloth on the skin to reduce irritation and close the pores.

13.   VAGINAL DOUCHING

Vaginal douching is basically washing your vagina from inside using water or other vaginal fluids. So, the question is whether or not vaginal douching is necessary for a healthy and clean vagina? No! it's so not necessary because your vagina is totally capable of cleaning itself and getting rid of harmful bacteria and dead cells. Your vagina produces glycogen which along with discharge, dead bad bacteria and worn out cells of your vaginal lining gets removed from the body.

Many women believe that regular vaginal douching is very essential to maintain a healthy vagina free from infections and bad odor. Little do they know, that vaginal douching is actually making them more prone to the infection. Once you clean your vagina, it may also lose its healthy bacteria and as soon as your guard is down bad bacteria will start to overpower good ones. Good bacterial species such as lactobacilli are responsible for the maintenance of vaginal ph. Once your vaginal pH goes out of balance, you're at the risk of getting infected with vaginal infections.

14. NEVER ENDING BENEFITS OF ACTIVATED CHARCOAL

Activated charcoal is basically finely ground black powder. It is made by heating the carbon powder or by treating it chemically. The process of heating or treating it makes it absorptive. It can absorb dirt, poisons and more. Activated charcoal is gaining more and more popularity due to its multiple health and beauty benefits. Let's discuss a few of its proven health and beauty benefits.

One of the most common uses of activated charcoal is teeth whitening and maintenance of oral health. Many toothpaste brands especially mention "with added activated charcoal". Its absorptive powers allow it to absorb dirt, plaque and can make your mouth bacteria free. It can be directly applied using toothbrush every day.

When used as a face mask or in a face mask it can absorb all the microparticles, dust and impurities from the deep pores of your skin. Activated charcoal is also capable of absorbing gases and smell, so it can also be used as a deodorant when applied in under arms or in your shoes. Medically it is used to remove the poisons and toxins from your body and also to treat overdosage of certain drugs.

15. MAINTAINING NAIL HYGIENE

As we all know, nail art is trending all over the globe these days. You can see a number of different ads offering unique, hot or cute nail art designs for all the occasions. There's no doubt that they make you look extremely elegant and classy but having longer nails might invite infections and germs too. Problems such as bacterial infections, fungal infections such as athlete's foot, food poisoning arise especially when you have long nails and you do not like to trim them or sometimes clean them properly.

The best way to clean your nails is to start with removing the dirt which is stuck underneath your nails. You can use nail pick for this purpose. Then wash your hands properly, not just your nails. Now that the dirt has been removed, hands have been washed, take some appropriately warm water not too hot nor too lukewarm and soak your nails in it for at least 10-15 minutes. You can also use a nail brush to scrub the tops slightly and make them look shiny and white.

Another method is to take baking soda or whitening toothpaste and mix it with hydrogen peroxide and scrub the top of your nails and underneath your nails lightly. Bleaching properties of these agents will whiten your nails, remove any unwanted germs or bacteria and makes them look shinier.

16. PROBIOTICS ARE YOUR BEST FRIEND!

The human body is home to a large number of microbes which naturally reside in your body, or on your skin. These microbes outnumber human body cells by 10:1, meaning for each human body cell there are 10 microbial cells. These microbes include bacteria, fungi and more and their function is to control the growth of bad bacteria in your system, kill them if they ever try to outnumber these good ones, protect your body from infections, improve your digestion and boost your immune function so that your body keeps functioning properly and maintain good health.

Sometimes due to unhealthy eating habits, unhygienic lifestyle and other causes, the natural balance of probiotics i.e. beneficial microorganisms is disturbed.

In order to restore the microbial flora of your gut and other organs, probiotics can be taken in the form of supplements, pills, dairy products or naturally from foods such as kefir, miso, pickles and more.

Probiotics contain different strains of healthy bacteria such as Bifidobacterium, Lactobacilli and few strains of yeast such a Saccharomyces Boulardii. All these beneficial microbes combine their powers and help in retaining the balance of the body.

17. NAIL YOUR WIPING TECHNIQUE

No matter how old you are or what you like to do with your genitals, the question to ask is this: are you serious about your hygiene? For example, you've been wiping for years after going to the toilets, so it's safe to say that you're an expert, right? Not necessarily! This is because many people may not know the perfect wiping technique.

One common problem that arises is cystitis causing UTIs in your urethra – the hole that you pee through. This is indeed one annoying problem which may cause you further pain and damage if not taken care of. A research conducted in Santa Barbara University, the right way to wipe is from top to bottom and not the other way around. If you are already doing this the right way, then you're good to go but it's time to get used to the right wiping technique if you used to do it the wrong way.

18.   AVOID SOAP TO MAINTAIN PH BALANCE

As you all might know that vagina is a sensitive and delicate area, something not to be messed with. But did you know that if your vagina's pH isn't steady, TSS can set in easily and quickly? Yes! That's true and even a researcher at Yale University has proven that lately.

The key is to avoid the excessive use of soap if you want to keep everything fresh. Just steer clear of them because most of the soaps can disturb your vaginal ph. Not just that but soaps are also capable of washing away what we call 'friendly' bacterium called lactobacilli. These friendly bacteria are something that helps keep the vagina its idea pH level (3.8 – 4.5) Also, lactobacilli are also very useful in combating bad bacteria such as S. aureus and other bad invaders as well.

So, what do you use when soap isn't an option anymore? Water. Just wash your vagina with water as its neutral pH works its way to keeping the lactobacilli happy which results in a healthy vagina.

19. BRUSH YOUR TONGUE

No matter if you brush your teeth twice a day or even sneak in for brush after lunch, chances are that if you don't start cleaning your tongue, you won't get rid of bad breath or lingering halitosis. Cleaning your tongue is not difficult as most toothbrushes come with a built-in tongue cleaner on the back. Food particles and bacteria are stored at the tongue under a thin layer of mucus. Use a small dab of toothpaste and start by brushing the top of the tongue and reach the back before working forward toward the opening of the mouth.

If you want to save all that trouble, then a tongue scrape may come in handy for you. It is made of soft and flexible plastic which easily peels the thin mucus-based layer from the tongue upon rinsing. Work slowly and apply light pressure or your tongue may start feeling sore or even bleed if too much pressure is applied. Cleaning your tongue regularly will not only rid you of bad breath but will also contribute to your overall hygiene.

20. LET'S WEAR COTTON UNDERWEAR

What's the first thing you consider when shopping or underwear? The cuts? The fabric? The feel? Sure, there are plenty of fancy and sexy underwear in their market but have you thought about choosing the one geared towards the well-being of the one who's wearing it?

Make sure that your underwear is not too tight because it would create discomfort when worn for long periods. Moreover, it limits the airflow to your vagina and that renders it as a bad option. The solution to all these problems is a regular fit cotton underwear which is best for its breathability. Also, make sure to not settle for anything less than 100% cotton – as they are available easily when shopping. Since the vagina is a self-cleaning organ, you have to allow the airflow for this to happen. Covering it with different materials that absorb moisture would create a room for bacteria to live.

21. TREAT INFECTIONS WHEN THEY ARISE

The monthly period not only brings pain and discomfort but it is also the time of the month when you are most prone to getting bacterial infections "down there". This is because menstrual periods increase your pH levels as blood is highly alkaline in nature. This is how the risk of an infection is increased.

Proper measures should be taken to be on a safe side, especially during these days. The use of "feminine wash" is recommended as they are formulated especially for such days. During the menstrual periods, it is recommended to wash "down there" at least 2 times a day using the feminine wash. Look for changes, rashes or any scars that might appear around your vagina and consult a doctor to treat any possible infection in time.

22. USE ENOUGH LUBRICANT, BUT NOT PETROLEUM JELLY

Lubrication, no doubt, is a vital aspect of the intercourse. If there is no or little lubrication, not only the sex would hurt, it may cause some bacterial infections as well. Some women do not produce enough natural lubricant during the intercourse of foreplay, so it is a good idea to use an artificial lubricant to reduce pain and enhance pleasure. However, one common misconception is the use of petroleum jelly as a lubricant. This is because products like petroleum jelly or baby oil are likely to cause inflammation or infections in women.

Go for the water or silicone-based lubes for increasing lubrication and make sure you use it before sex even happens. Another idea is to use it inside a condom, to be on a safe side. Not only it would reduce the risk of a possible infection, but it would also enhance the pleasure, thanks to the added lubrication by you.

23.   EATING AND HYGIENE

Chances are you have read hundreds of blog posts and tried countless diet plans but nothing really worked to perfection, eh? We're not talking about all that but rather our focus is on 'clean eating' both in terms of being hygienic and healthy. Ensure that you wash your hands every time to prevent cross-contamination (which ultimately results in food poisoning). Whether you are cooking for yourself or someone else, make sure that food or anything that comes in contact with food does not touch your body or anything you are wearing.

Other steps include washing your hands immediately after handling raw foods such as eggs and meat etc., touching pets or going to the toilet. Keep the pet's food away from cooked food and anything edible at your place. Also, many people don't take notice but it is recommended to keep the pets away from your food and food preparing and eating areas. Pets are more likely to pass on an infection than anything else.

24.   URINATE AFTER SEX

Being a woman, chances are that you must have heard about it a lot! Peeing after having sex. Urinating after sex is one of those rules that all women dutifully follow, or knowingly ignore. Surely, no woman wants to get UTI (Urinary tract infection). According to doctors, sex is commonly associated with UTIs because, in this process, bacteria is introduced through the urethra and ultimately into a woman's urinary tract.

When you pee after having sex, it helps greatly in flushing out the bacteria BEFORE they can gather up in the bladder. Of course, you don't have to have a stopwatch or you don't have to jump out of your bed right after having sex. You just have to make sure that you go to the washroom before you fall asleep – which is a probable case after having sex. Also, don't ever hold the pee – if you are having the urge to urinate any time of the day, do not ignore it.

25.   INCLUDE MORE YOGURT IN YOUR DIET

You know how the saying goes, "A bowl of yogurt a day, keeps diseases at bay". This is for a reason because there are lots of proteins, zinc, calcium, and potassium in yogurt along with vitamin B12. As a research by Nutrition Research in 2013 states that women who consume yogurt on regular basis have a healthier diet than those who don't.

Having yogurt on daily basis is commonly associated with lower blood pressure and glucose level in blood. Also, less insulin resistance results in lower chances of catching chronic diseases. One of the most useful advantages of yogurt is in dieting; since it is full of protein, consuming yogurt on regular basis may help you control your calories intake. Thus, you are able to achieve a better weight management and better organize your calorie intake.

Apart from all the aforementioned benefits, consistent consumption of yogurt also reduces the possibility of a nutrient deficiency in women. Overall, yogurt contributes to you enjoying a healthier lifestyle and there's no reason why you should not make it a part of your meal.

26. GET REGULAR TESTING FOR STDS

It is a common misconception which makes people think that they would know if they had an STD (Sexually transmitted disease). Wrong! The reality is that there are no signs or symptoms in most of the STD cases. Even the symptoms that are shown are mild, and thus can be easily overlooked or confused with something else. Hence, you may have heard the new term STI (sexually transmitted infection); the only way to know for sure is to get tested.

A lot of women have a presumption that their annual medical check-up includes STI tests. This may or may not be the case, so make sure that you ask for it. Especially if you have had more than one sex partners or had unprotected sex, it is a must to know for sure and gets tested as soon as possible.

Get in touch with your healthcare provider or a clinic near you and develop a habit of getting tested or STIs on regular basis.

27.   MILD SOAPS TO WASH THE BREAST AREA

Your choice of soap may as well result in pimples on your face and breasts. While they don't usually pose a major health risk, they sure are uncomfortable and it is easy to treat them. Remember, all you have to do to treat a breast pimple and rashes to change certain habits and use OTC medications. There are plenty of home treatments and minor changes in lifestyle that would greatly help in curing the pimples. If you have developed breast pimples, make sure to wash the area regularly with mild soap, twice a day.

If you have long hair and especially if it reaches your chest, it could very well be a reason contributing to pimples. Develop a habit of washing your hair if it feels oily. Also, it is easy to sit back and relax on a couch after a workout routine and let the sweat dry off. What you may not know is that sweat is also known to produce pimples if not showered within a reasonable time.

If you want to step up and stick to applying something on your skin to cure acne, go for tea tree oil. It comes in the form of gel or wash and might cure your pimples.

28.   CONSIDER TAKING LIQUID CHLOROPHYLL

Don't let the name startle you and it is perfectly fine if it's the first time you are reading about it. Chlorophyll is naturally present in the green vegetables and is known to be a great health supplement. There are several studies that prove great benefits of chlorophyll on skin, body odors and also for treating certain types of cancer.

If you are a working woman or your lifestyle involves going outside and getting exposed to sunlight, chlorophyll might come in handy. This is because chlorophyll gel reduces photoaging – the aging as a result of sun exposure. Besides that, chlorophyll gel is also greatly beneficial for curing acne and pores.

Besides having benefits for skin, chlorophyll also has blood-building properties as you can add a glass of wheatgrass juice that helps to treat a number of hemoglobin deficiency disorders.

Last but not least, one irresistible property of chlorophyll is weight loss! According to researchers, including green plant membrane supplement once per day in your diet not only reduces the urge to eat but also encourages weight loss.

29.   FLOSS!

Accept it or not: flossing really does matter. Not only for the protection and good health and teeth and gums but flossing also confers several other benefits. The important thing to know is that it is more about removing the dental plaque rather than just removing the food debris. It is the complicated bacterial ecosystem that is developed between the teeth and it is responsible for causing tooth decay, periodontal disease, and several other related problems.

Start flossing to preserve your teeth and to keep the aesthetics of your smile. Almost all of the floss is made of either nylon or Teflon and both are equally effective. If your teeth are close together, without much spaces in between, thin floss might work a lot better for you. There are chances that you would see a little bit of blood but don't worry, it only means that the gums are inflamed thanks to the plaque, which needs to be cleaned ASAP.

30.   GET TO KNOW YOUR VAGINAL SCENT

Let's cut to the chase: Have you ever wondered about the natural smell of your vagina? As you may know, the vagina is supposed to have a specific smell, which varies for every woman. However, it is normal to have unusual vaginal odors, even if you are taking good care of your body. The key is to get to know your natural vaginal scent. After the menstrual period, the bad smell is likely to last for a few days but it is the persistence of bad odor that is the problem.

The first in line about what you should change in your lifestyle to get rid of these bad odors is stay away from perfumes soaps and body washes. What you may not know is that vagina is capable of self-cleaning and maintaining its pH on its own. Using different kinds of cosmetic products like body washes and perfumed soaps disturbs the natural pH of the vagina. Another good idea would be to change your underwear if you currently use silk, satin or polyester panties and stick to the only cotton. It lets your vagina breathe, stay fresh and free from odors.

31. CORRECT CLEANSER FOR YOUR SKIN TYPE

We all know that basic skincare starts with a good cleansing session. Any good cleanser will be gentle, irritant-free and won't leave your skin dry and sticky after a thorough rinsing. However, it is important to know which cleanser suits your skin type and we will help you choose one.

If you have oily skin then you should be looking for an oil-free facewash capable of digging deep for a through pore cleaning. Also, go for the one with charcoal which has great properties and helps in controlling the oil production without making your face too dry.

Gel cleansers is a good choice if you prefer hydrating products that are lightweight. They are good for gently removing the makeup, moisturizing the skin and rejuvenate it to give you a fresh look and feel. Such cleansers are a good choice for normal to a bit oily skin.

If you are the kind of woman who likes to use cotton pads for removing makeup, micellar water is the one to go for. Shake them up really good before use and they would remove any makeup without leaving any greasy layer on your face.

32.   GENTLE EXFOLIATION TWICE A WEEK

Over-exfoliation is one of those mistakes that almost all of us women make. Exfoliating too much with a hard scrub may backfire big time so it is important to know how often you should exfoliate. The bottom line is that more than 3 to 4 times a week is too much, regardless of what skin type or the lifestyle you have.

Anything more than that is likely to create small cracks in your skin to worsen your looks.

Also, make sure that you are gentle while exfoliating and don't torture your skin like it has some secret government information. Go for a scrub with sugar crystals because they are able to dissolve your dead skin cells without too much irritation. Since you cannot exfoliate every day, what you can do is use Salicylic acid as a cleanser and also as an oil-control agent.

33. STAY HYDRATED

Ladies! Sweating is critical for your keeping your body temperature regulated. However, if you are involved in some sort of workout routine, then keeping yourself hydrated is very important not only for your body but also for brain functions. Also, if you suffer from occasional headaches, it is most likely because of insufficient water intake. Apart from that, drinking lots and lots of water also helps in relieving constipation and treat kidney stones naturally.

Make sure that you are getting 6 to 8 glasses of water every day to stay in good shape and enjoy a healthier and rejuvenated skin. That's true because it is water that keeps your muscles lubricated and energized as you work out. Last but not least and the most overlooked benefit of drinking lots of water: weight loss. Drinking water increases your satiety and enhances your metabolism.

34.   GET ENOUGH SLEEP

Between work life, workout routine, social life and a bit of personal space, many women do not enough sleep. It is important to note that sleep affects your mental and physical health and it is up to you whether you'd want a positive or negative effect. Also, women are more likely to have insomnia than men as menstrual periods, pregnancy and other factors affect strongly on how a woman sleep.

Did you know that your body and your brain work best when you are in a state of complete rest i.e. asleep? However, if you are having trouble sleeping and are unable to determine the reason, you may consider talking to your doctor to prescribe you some over-the-counter (OTC) medicines to help you asleep. It is easy to fall prey to insomnia when taking too much stress from anything. However, indulging in activities such as yoga, meditating and praying often helps in getting a good night's sleep. Getting at least 7 to 8 hours of sleep every day is vital for your health.

35. MAKE SUNSCREENS YOUR BEST FRIEND

Sunscreens are the most neglected and ignored essentials. Most of the girls don't even consider buying it when they're shopping for beauty or health care products. Well trust me, you don't want to go out on a sunny day without a sunscreen. Wish to know why? This is because the sun has rays called ultraviolet rays (UVA and UVB), these rays are capable of penetrating your skin deep. Their penetration might cause infections, increased production of melatonin which can darken your skin tone and can even cause skin cancer!!

Sunscreens have sun protection factor or SPF value mentioned on them. Usually, dermatologist suggests applying SPF-15 evenly on your skin with a reasonably thick layer but if you wish to stay protected without applying a thicker layer you can opt for SPF-30. SPF-15 provides 93% protection from UVB rays and SPF-30 provides 97% protection. If the nature of your job or hobby makes you stay out under the open sun, you should keep your exposed body parts covered with sunscreen and reapply it after every two hours. That will do the trick.

36. MOISTURIZING YOUR SKIN

If your skin feels like a sandpaper and appears to be dead, flaky or cracking then you really need to step up your moisturizing games. Some of us might have naturally dry skin, while others get to have it as an added perk of the winter season. In either case, your skin needs total inside out moisturizing. It doesn't mean that you can apply a ton of moisturizing lotion and be done with it. A complete skin care routine and a set of healthy habits are needed to make sure that your skin is glowing and hydrated.

First of all, you need to develop a habit of drinking more than 8 glasses of water per day. Your body is 70% water and a hydrated body means a hydrated and healthy skin. Food items such as spinach, nuts, whole grains, and salmon have omega-3, vitamin C and Vitamin E in them. Adding them in your diet might naturally boost your skin, keep it hydrated and will make it look healthy and supple. Now that you have taken care of your dietary and water intake. It's time to maintain a healthy skin care routine. Adding a few drops of essential oils such as lavender or tea tree in your bathtub will keep infections and dead skin at bay. Make sure to reduce your bath time and use water which is lukewarm and not too hot. Lastly, apply moisturizing lotions or creams which suits your skin on your body right after taking a bath.

37.   HAIR CARE ROUTINE

Your hair needs a routine of their own to keep them healthy and shining and it includes washing, drying, styling, night time and daytime routines. That might sound hectic but you don't get anything for free, you have got to invest in your hair but fortunately some time and effort, not your money.

 If you struggle from a lot of bad hair days then its high time you start to oil them at least before washing. Apply any oil you like such as olive oil or coconut oil at least half an hour before taking a shower and voila! you have naturally conditioned hair. First of all, don't shower too often and if you have to, then make sure to dilute your shampoo with a mug of water. Avoid using hot water to wash your hair, it might damage them. Try drying your hair with a microfiber towel and comb them when they're still wet, this way your hair will not get tangled.

You can also apply hair mask at least twice or thrice a month to give them an extra boost. Take a fully ripe banana, add it into the blender. Blend it with few drops of lemon, any oil, and honey. Make a paste out of it, apply this paste evenly on your hair tips, not the scalp or roots. Rinse your hair with lukewarm warm water after 20-30 minutes and enjoy silky soft and shinier hair.

38.   EAT YOUR GREENS!

Many mums struggle with their kids especially when it comes to making them eat vegetables. Not just kids, most of the grown-ups would also like to avoid green vegetables. What if I tell you these unappealing leafy green vegetables are just what you need to maintain a beautiful skin and body! Firstly, they are rich in fibers and minerals which help in digestion. They don't allow your food to stay in your gut for longer duration and hence they aid in reducing the weight too. Green vegetables reduce the amount of blood sugar and your chances of getting diabetes too.

They are also rich in Vitamin C and antioxidants which help in boosting your immunity, avoiding the infections, keeping you active and delay the process of aging. Their high calcium content helps in maintaining bone and teeth health. The green vegetables have a high content of iron and folate which prevent your body from heart problems

39.   GREEN TEA FOR WEIGHT LOSS

If you're interested to lose some pounds and don't know exactly from where to start then simply try adding few cups of green tea in your diet along with some exercises. Green tea has a wide range of health benefits. Most importantly they improve digestion and metabolism. They have catechin an antioxidant which is responsible for boosting your metabolism, a process by which you convert your food into energy. Improved metabolism ultimately helps in reducing weight. Catechin also speeds up the process of breaking of fats into usable energy, furthermore, caffeine present in them also boosts it weight loss properties.

Other health benefits of green tea include reduced risk of heart problems, relieving stress and keeping you light and beautiful.

40. DARK COLORED UNDERGARMENTS AND CANCER

Most people consider it a myth that dark-colored undergarments increase your chances of getting cancer. Let's talk about it logically.

Basically, the thing is dark colors such as black absorb more visible light and when it doesn't reflect anything back it appears to be black. Now when it comes to black underwear or bras, they work in the same way i.e. they absorb more rays and light from the sun. Sun rays are accompanied by ultraviolet rays such as UVA and UVB rays. These rays are capable of penetrating into the skin and speed up the process of aging, causing sunburn and more. Once they penetrate into the skin, they are capable of causing mutations and ultimately cancer! Make sure that you wear light colored bras mostly and also allow your body to breathe by not wearing bras at night or wearing loose undergarments.

41. DEALING WITH THE AFTER-EFFECTS OF VAGINAL BIRTH

Giving a vaginal birth might be difficult and painful but dealing with the tender, achy, swollen lady parts, those sutures you got and heavy bleeding is a whole new story.

First things first, switch to healthier foods. This includes taking hard boiled eggs and a cup of warm milk with a pinch of turmeric to reduce inflammation and pain. Food rich in fibers will improve your metabolism and digestion. Drinking lukewarm water will also help to reduce swelling and will soothe your body. Now that you have enjoyed 9 period-free months, it's time to deal with the heaviest bleeding ever, for this purpose you can take two pads at a time or you can put them side by side. While pooping, try not to strain too much and taking laxatives is actually a good practice. Try wiping with a medicated pad because you don't want to get any bacterial infection.

Lastly, cold presses can also help a great deal in soothing the tenderness.

42.   GOODBYE CHAPPED LIPS

Drinks such as coffee, tea and alcohol and extreme weather conditions of your country might make your lips all chapped and flaky. If you want to keep them plump, healthy and hydrated you simply need to follow these steps. First of all, cover them with lip balm before washing your face with a face wash. Drink lots and lots of water. Exfoliate them gently with your toothbrush and warm water to remove the dead flakes, then apply lip balm. Try looking for ingredients such as shea butter, macadamia oil, and honey in your lip products. Sunburn can also cause a severe damage to your lips so apply sunscreen every time you move out of your house. You can also apply glycerin and rose water in the proportion 1:1 on your lips every night, this will keep them hydrated and moisturized.

43.   REMOVING BLACKHEADS

Blackheads are formed when the pores on your face get clogged with dirt, sebum and dead skin cell. Once the pores are clogged their surface remains open and due to the process of oxidation, they appear to be black. Removing these unwanted and unappealing tiny black dots can be a bit tricky. Starting from your cleansing routine, make sure that you wash your face at least twice or thrice a day so that dirt and mud won't clog your pores. It is advisable to use face wash that contain salicylic acid, it helps in breaking down the particles which are clogging the pores. If you wish to remove them at home with a steel or plastic blackhead remover, make sure they're properly sterilized. Then take a steamy bath or wash your face with warm water to open up the pores. Once your pores loosen up a bit, then try using your blackhead removing tool but don't go hard on your skin.

44.   TREATING YOUR CRACKED HEELS

The most neglected part of your body in most of the cases are your feet. They have to bear the weight of your whole body and they're the ones dealing with all the dirt, puddles and harsh conditions. Lack of proper care makes them dull and your heels cracked.

 In order to heal the cracks in your heels and preventing them from cracking again soak your feet in lukewarm water for 20-30 minutes. Scrub them and exfoliate them gently with a loofah and a foot cleanser. Once you've cleaned your feet properly, try dipping them in warm water again and this time add few drops of oil and glycerin in the water. Massage them gently. Dry them with a soft towel and apply moisturizer on them. Wear socks and change them daily to avoid getting and infections and bad odor.

45. LONGER LASHES MAKE YOU MORE BEAUTIFUL

Who doesn't want to have long and dramatic lashes? If you're seeking ways to enhance the natural beauty of your lashes and give them an extra volume then simply add following remedies to your everyday routine. For the first natural remedy, you can take an empty mascara bottle and fill it with some castor oil and olive oil (equal parts), shake it well, apply this mixture on your lashes every night before going to bed. Leave it on till morning and wash your face like you normally do the next morning. Another way to enhance the growth of your lashes includes applying petroleum jelly directly on your lashes every night before going to bed.

Last but not least, you can also take shea butter and mix a capsule of Vitamin E with it (equal parts) and massage it on the roots of the lashes gently. Leave it on for the night, you can do this until you see visible results.

46.   BEST DETOXIFIERS!

Your body has a natural detoxifying system which keeps it free from toxins and build-up of unhealthy and unwanted substances in the body. Occasionally, due to overexposure to extreme conditions, unhealthy eating and sedentary lifestyle might mess with your natural detox system. This is the point where an extra helping hand won't hurt. Following are some of the best detoxifiers that will do the trick.

Grapefruit juice is known for its multiple health benefits. It reduces cholesterol level, flavonoids present in it can repair tissue damage associated with diabetic complications, and it can boost your immunity too. Garlic and ginger both have strong antioxidant and detoxifying properties owing to the flavonoids and organosulfur compounds present in them. Other examples of natural detoxifiers include cabbage, beets and more.

47. BEAUTY BENEFITS OF TURMERIC

Turmeric, a natural spice, is known for centuries for its extremely beneficial health and beauty effects. Curcumin a chemical ingredient present in it is actually responsible for all its antioxidant and anti-inflammatory properties. Turmeric is widely used for its antioxidant, anti-infective, antiseptic and anti-inflammatory properties.

Drinking a cup of warm milk with few a teaspoonful of turmeric powder might help you boost your immunity because curcumin fight the free radicals present in your body. Turmeric is also known for its skin lightening properties. Make a paste out of milk and turmeric and apply it on your face, it will reduce the production of melanin, a pigment responsible for the darkening of the skin. It also has strong antiseptic and anti-infective properties, therefore, gentle exfoliation with turmeric powder and rose water will reduce the chances of acne burst out.

48. MINTY FRESH BREATH

Nobody wants to be in an embarrassing situation where they don't even know that their breath is smelling bad and people are trying to avoid them.

Certain foods can make your mouth smell bad, commonly garlic, onions, and ginger are blamed for it. They have a number of organosulfur compounds which can give a characteristic odor to your breath. Make sure to wash your mouth with a mouthwash every time you eat any of these. While brushing your teeth, brush your tongue and internal lining of your mouth too. It will help in removing debris and bad bacteria from the mouth too. Furthermore, drinking lots of water will also help to wash away all the bad odor-causing bacteria. Finally, add parsley and mint in your smoothies and meal, they have antibacterial properties and above that, they give your mouth a fresh minty fragrance.

49. REMOVE YOUR SUNTAN

Natural tanning is basically your body's way of defending itself from the harmful UV radiations. When your body is exposed to the sun for longer durations, a pigment called melanin start to build up in your skin making it look darker in appearance. The problem is it can give you uneven skin tone, areas which remain covered will appear lighter in tone and exposed areas will appear darker. You all know that removing a tan is not like taking a body wash and scrubbing it off, it is a lot more difficult. Follow this tan removing technique in order to get rid of its uneven skin tone. Start with cleansing the affected parts with lemon and milk. Bleaching properties of lemon will help in lightening the skin tone. Once you have cleansed the affected parts, take a bowl and add coconut oil, brown sugar, turmeric, and Aloe Vera to it. Mix the ingredients well, gently exfoliate the skin with this mixture, then let it dry and scrub the remaining mixture off. Finally, wash the area with warm water and apply a soothing moisturizer. Repeat this twice a week and see for yourself, the magic of this natural tan removing wonder.

50.   SAY NO TO FRIZZY HAIR

Excessive use of hair dryers, hair straighteners and curlers, dehydration and washing your hair more often with shampoos can make them dull and frizzy. If you have frizzy hair that doesn't necessarily mean that the natural texture of your hair is frizzy, it might also mean that you're not keeping your hair naturally nourished and moisturized. Following are some of the best combo remedies to prevent frizzy hair. Eggs and almond oil, coconut oil and Vitamin E, lemon and honey with few drops of apple cider vinegar. You simply have to choose your favorite combo and mix them together. Apply them on your hair at least twice a week and leave them on for 20-30 minutes. Then wash them off with tap water and you're good to go. All these ingredients have natural hair conditioning, nourishing and moisturizing properties.

OTHER HELPFUL RESOURCES

- WebMD. https://www.webmd.com/

- Healthline. https://www.healthline.com/

- WikiHow.
  https://www.wikihow.com/Main-Page

READ OTHER

50 THINGS TO KNOW

BOOKS

50 Things to Know

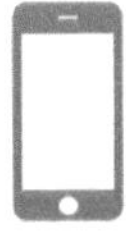

Website: 50thingstoknow.com

Facebook: facebook.com/50thingstoknow

Pinterest: pinterest.com/lbrennec

YouTube: youtube.com/user/50ThingsToKnow

Twitter: twitter.com/50ttk

Mailing List: Join the 50 Things to Know
Mailing List to Learn About New Releases

50 Things to Know

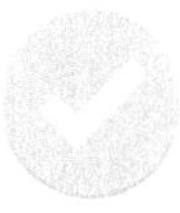

Please leave your honest review of this book on Amazon and Goodreads. We appreciate your positive and constructive feedback. Thank you.

www.ingramcontent.com/pod-product-compliance
Lightning Source LLC
Chambersburg PA
CBHW051226250726
48655CB00006B/2631